My Mediterranean Cooking Guide

An Unmissable Collection of Avocado, Chicken, Soup Recipes & Much More

Marta Jackson

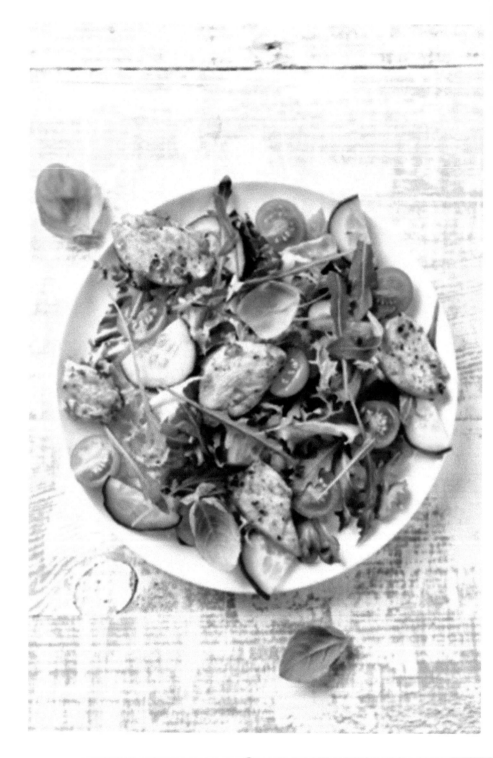

Table of Contents

Garden glut soup

Ingredients

- 1 organic vegetable stock cube
- 1 medium onion
- 100g of podded fresh peas
- A2 sticks of celery
- a few sprigs of fresh mint
- 1 medium leek
- 200g of baby spinach
- 2 cloves of garlic
- Olive oil
- 3 medium potatoes

Directions

- Combine chopped onion, celery, garlic, and leek in a small bowel.
- Place a large pot on a medium heat with 2 tablespoons of olive oil.
- When hot, add vegetables the in the small bowl, lower the heat and cook with the lid askew for 10 to 15 minutes, stirring occasionally.

- Place chopped potatoes, courgette in a bowl.
- Fill and boil the kettle.
- Add the potatoes, courgettes, once the vegetables are cooked, with a tiny pinch of sea salt and black pepper.
- Crumble the stock cube into a measuring jug.
- Top up the boiling water and stir until dissolved.
- Pour the hot stock into the pot.
- Raise the heat to high and bring to the boil.
- Cook over low heat for 15 to 20 minutes or until the potato is cooked through.
- Add the peas with spinach and cook for 4 more minutes.
- Remove the pot to a heatproof surface, let rest.
- Blend until smooth.
- Ladle the soup into bowls and sprinkle over the mint.
- Serve and enjoy.

Asian noodles broth with fish

Ingredients

- 2 fresh red chilies
- 250g of fresh egg noodles
- 2 limes, juice
- Sea salt
- Low-salt soy sauce
- 220g can of water shell nuts
- Freshly ground black pepper
- Sesame oil
- Vegetable oil
- 2 cloves garlic
- 1 small bunch fresh coriander
- 1 thumb-sized piece of fresh ginger
- 100g of mange tout
- 1 liter of organic fish
- 500g of sole fillets

Directions

- Bring a pan of salted water to the boil.
- Place in and cook the noodles as instructed on the pack.

- Drain the noodles in a colander, toss in a little sesame oil.
- Divide the noodles between four serving bowls.
- Heat a large frying pan over a medium heat.
- Add a splash of vegetable oil.
- Stir-fry the garlic together with the ginger, mange tout, water shell nuts, and half the chilies for 2 minutes.
- Add the hot stock and bring to the boil.
- Place in the sole pieces, cook for a minute.
- Season generously with soy sauce and black pepper.
- Serve and enjoy.

Brown Windsor soup with pearl barley

Ingredients

- 1 tablespoon of plain flour
- 1 large knob of unsalted butter
- Olive oil
- 2 liters of organic beef stock
- 1 fresh bay leaf
- 500g of diced stewing steak
- 1 tablespoon of Marmite
- 2 carrots
- 150g of pearl barley
- 1 splash of Worcestershire sauce
- 1 sprig of fresh rosemary
- 1 red onion
- 3 sticks of celery

Directions

- Melt the butter in a large pan over a medium heat.
- Add a splash of olive oil with the steak, and lightly brown the meat.

- Stir in the Marmite with the Worcestershire sauce.
- Raise the heat to high and keep stirring until all the liquid has evaporated.
- Add carrots together with the onions, bay leaf, rosemary sprig, and celery, cook over a low heat covered until soft.
- Stir in the flour, pour in the stock.
- Season well with sea salt and black pepper.
- Bring to the boil, lower the heat to let simmer.
- Add the pearl barley, let cook gently for 1 hour.
- Remove, then discard the rosemary sprig with bay leaf.
- Whisk the soup to thicken.
- Serve and enjoy with hunks of soda bread.

Chicken garden soup

Ingredients

- A few sprigs of fresh flat-leaf parsley
- 2 onions
- 200g of baby spinach
- 6 carrots
- 2 handfuls of seasonal greens
- 6 sticks of celery
- 1 lemon
- 1 large knob of unsalted butter
- 2 fresh bay leaves
- 4 shallots
- 4 whole peppercorns
- 2 cloves of garlic
- 1 free-range of roast chicken carcass
- Olive oil

Directions

- Put chopped onions, carrots, celery, bay leaves, peppercorns, chicken carcass, and a pinch of salt in a bowl.

- Fill the pan with cold water, then place on a high heat and bring to the boil.
- Lower the heat, let a simmer and cook for 1 hour, skimming off any scum.
- About 20 minutes before the stock is ready, crack on with the base of the soup.
- Place the butter with 1 tablespoon of oil in a separate large pan on a low heat.
- Add the garlic together with the shallots and parsley stalks, let cook for 10 minutes.
- Add the carrots with celery, cook for a further 5 minutes.
- When the stock is ready, remove the chicken carcass with any remaining pieces of meat and leave to one side. Throw the carcass.
- Strain the stock through a sieve into the veggie pan.
- Bring to the boil, then reduce heat, simmer for 20 minutes.
- Add the seasonal greens, cook for 10 minutes.
- Add the spinach in the last minute.

- Divide between bowls and top with any leftover shredded chicken.
- Serve and enjoy sprinkled with parsley leaves and black pepper.

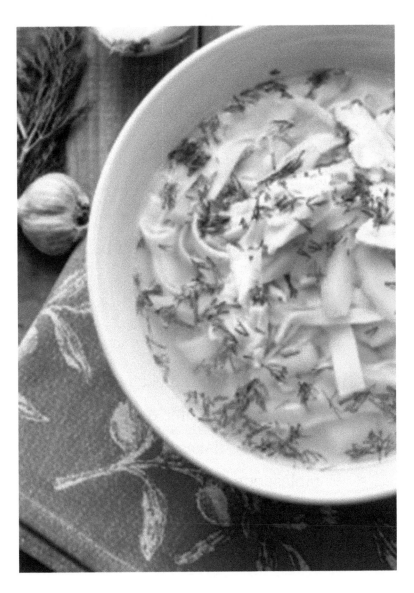

Chunky squash and chickpea soup

Ingredients

- 1 dried red chili
- Sea salt
- A few sprigs of fresh mint
- Olive oil
- 2 sticks celery
- 1 tablespoon of cumin seeds
- Harissa paste
- 2 lemons, zest
- 3 cloves garlic
- A few sprigs of fresh flat-leaf parsley
- 1 butternut squash
- 2 small red onions
- Extra virgin olive oil
- 1.5 liters of organic chicken
- 2 x 400g of tinned chickpeas
- 50g of almond flakes
- ½ tablespoon of fennel seeds
- ½ tablespoon of sesame seeds
- ½ tablespoon of poppy seeds

- Freshly ground black pepper

Directions

- Begin by preheating your oven ready to 400°F.
- Place the squash together with the cumin, and crumbled chili on to a baking tray.
- Drizzle with olive oil, mix together and place in the preheated oven.
- Roast for 45 minutes until the squash is cooked through.
- Heat a large saucepan once the squash is roasted, pour in a splash of oil.
- Add the celery together with the garlic, parsley stalks, and 2/3 of the onion, cook gently until softened, covered.
- Place in the roasted squash and let it sweat for a few minutes
- Pour in the stock. Bring to the boil.
- Let simmer for 15 minutes over low heat.
- Add the chickpeas and simmer for 15 minutes more.

- Toast the reserved squash seeds with the almond flakes, fennel, sesame, and poppy seeds in a little olive oil until all colored.
- Season, then blend briefly to thickens.
- Mix lemon zest together with the chopped parsley leaves, and mint leaves.
- Chop the remaining onion until it's really fine, add to zesty mixture, mix.
- Spoon half a teaspoon of harissa paste into each bowl.
- Divide the zesty herb mixture between the bowls and ladle over the soup.
- Stir each bowl with a spoon
- Serve and enjoy with the toasted seeds and almonds

Coconut millet bowl with berbere spiced squash and chickpeas

This is a plant based Mediterranean Sea diet that features shallots, spinach, millet grain, and coconut milk with vibrant flavors and spices.

Ingredients

- water
- 1 ½ lb. kabocha squash 3/4 slices
- 2 large shallots, sliced
- 1 cup of millet
- 1 teaspoon of grated fresh ginger
- 1 tablespoon of coconut oil
- ¼ cup of fresh mint leaves
- ¼ teaspoon of turmeric
- ¼ teaspoon salt
- ½ cup of fresh cilantro
- 15 oz. can chickpeas, drained
- 3 cups of fresh spinach
- ½ cup of coconut cream
- 2 tablespoons avocado oil
- ¼ cup of lime juice

- zest of one lime
- 1 teaspoon <u>honey</u>
- 2 tablespoons <u>Berbere spice</u>
- 1 cup of <u>coconut milk</u>
- ½ cup of cucumber chunks

Directions

- Set your oven to 400°F.
- Combine <u>berbere</u> , olive oil, and water in a bowl, hydrate for 10 minutes.
- Set aside some <u>coconut milk</u> .
- Boil the remaining <u>coconut milk</u> mixed with water, turmeric, and <u>salt</u> to a simmer.
- Add <u>coconut oil</u> with millet bring to a gentle boil, lower heat, let simmer for 15 minutes covered.
- Place prepared squash, shallots and chickpeas on <u>sheet pan</u> with <u>parchment</u> .
- Spread the <u>berbere</u> paste with a brush.
- Sprinkle with <u>salt</u> and place in oven for 30 minutes.

- Combine and blend the reserved coconut cream, <u>salt</u>, <u>honey</u>, cucumber, lime juice, and zest, and fresh ginger until smooth.
- Add the cilantro and mint, blend for few seconds.
- Assemble the bowls with the veggies on top of the warm millet.
- Then, add fresh spinach and drizzle with the sauce.
- Serve and enjoy.

Instant pot pinto bean stew

Ingredients

- 1 teaspoon of <u>chipotle powder</u>
- 2 teaspoons Molasses
- 1 tablespoon of olive oil
- 1 teaspoon of <u>salt</u>
- 1 large onion, chopped
- 4 cups of chopped poblano peppers
- 1 yam
- 4 cloves garlic coarsely chopped
- 14 oz. can of crushed tomatoes
- 3 cups of <u>veggie broth</u>
- 2 teaspoons of Ancho chili powder
- 1 cup of frozen corn
- 1 teaspoon of <u>cumin</u>
- 1 ½ cups of dry pinto beans
- 1 teaspoon of <u>coriander</u>

<u>Directions</u>

- Set instant pot to Sauté.
- Then, add olive oil with the onion, let sauté 5 minutes.

- Add garlic and poblanos continue to sauté for 2 minutes.
- Add the ancho chili powder together with the cumin, and coriander, stirring to coat.
- Add the yams together with soaked beans, molasses, chipotle, tomatoes, chicken stock, and salt .
- Set the Instant Pot to high pressure for 25 minutes.
- Manually release pressure valve.
- Stir in frozen corn and let warm through.
- Serve and enjoy.

Curried zucchini soup

Ingredients

- 2 teaspoons of <u>yellow curry powder</u>
- 2 tablespoons of <u>coconut oil</u>
- ¼ cup of cilantro- leaves
- 1 medium onion
- 2 cloves garlic
- 4 cups of chicken
- ¼ cup of mint leaves
- 1 tablespoon of ginger
- 1 jalapeño
- 1 ½ teaspoons of <u>sea salt</u>
- 2 pounds of zucchini or yellow squash

Directions

- In a heavy-bottomed pot sauté onion with garlic, ginger, and jalapeño in <u>coconut oil</u> , for 5 minutes over medium heat.
- Add the <u>salt</u> together with the zucchini and curry powder.
- Sauté briefly.
- Add 2 cups of the broth.

- Let simmer, covered and cook until the summer squash is tender.
- Add another 2 cups of cold broth to the <u>blender</u> with all the simmered ingredients.
- Blend, until smooth with a vented lid.
- Add fresh mint and cilantro, blend to incorporated.
- Serve and enjoy.

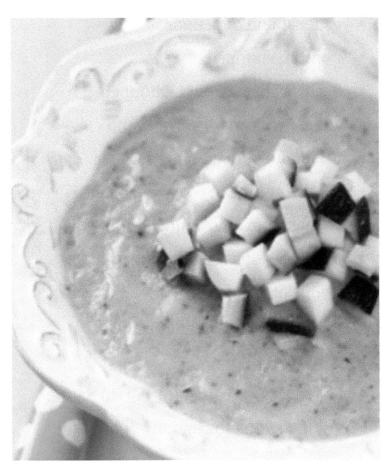

White bean chili with jackfruit

Ingredients

- 1 teaspoon of <u>salt</u>
- 1 tablespoon of <u>coriander</u>
- 1 tablespoon of <u>cumin</u>
- 2 tablespoons of <u>olive oil</u>
- 1 teaspoon of <u>sugar</u>
- 2 teaspoons of <u>granulated garlic</u>
- ½ teaspoon of pepper
- 1 onion, chopped
- 6 garlic cloves, rough chopped
- 2 teaspoons of <u>dried oregano</u>
- 1 poblano pepper, chopped
- 2 x 14-ounce cans of white beans
- ½ teaspoon of ground <u>chipotle powder</u>
- 16 ounces of canned <u>jackfruit</u>
- 3 cups of <u>veggie broth</u>
- 1 tablespoon of <u>chili powder</u>

<u>Directions</u>

- Firstly, set your <u>Instant Pot</u> to Sauté.
- Then, heat 2 tablespoons of olive oil.

- Add onion together with the garlic and fresh poblano, let sauté for 3 minutes until fragrant.
- Add canned chilies together with the canned beans and jackfruit .
- Add the veggie broth .
- Add all the spice along with sugar and salt .
- Stir and set Instant pot to a high heat for 10 minutes.
- Naturally release the pressure.
- Stir in corn with chopped kale and cover for 5 minutes on warm setting.
- Taste, and adjust the seasoning.
- Serve in bowls with diced avocado , cilantro, radishes.
- Serve and enjoy.

Moroccan red lentil quinoa soup

Ingredients

- 2 tablespoons of olive oil
- 1 teaspoon of maple syrup
- 1 teaspoon of dried thyme
- 1 teaspoon of coriander
- 1 onion, diced
- 3/4 cup of red lentils
- 6 garlic cloves, rough chopped
- 3 carrots, diced
- 1 red bell pepper, diced
- 1 teaspoon of cinnamon
- ¼ cup of quinoa
- 1 poblano pepper, diced
- 1 14-ounce can of diced tomatoes
- 4 cups veggie broth
- 1 ½ teaspoon of salt
- 2 teaspoons of cumin
- 1 teaspoon of chili powder
- ½ teaspoon of turmeric

Directions

- **Set** Instant Pot **to sauté function.**
- Heat olive oil.
- Then, sauté the onion and garlic for 4 minutes, stirring until fragrant.
- Add the carrots together with bell pepper, stir 2 minutes.
- Add the diced tomatoes and broth.
- Stir in the salt together with the cumin, chili powder, cinnamon, mable syrup, coriander, turmeric, and thyme .
- Stir in the split red lentils with the quinoa.
- Set instant pot to high pressure for 5 minutes.
- Manually release the pressure.
- Taste, and adjust the seasoning.
- Serve and enjoy with fresh radishes and herbs.

Potato wedges

Ingredients

- Olive oil
- Sea salt
- 600g of baking potatoes
- Freshly ground black pepper

Directions

- Firstly, preheat your oven ready to 400°F.
- Put a large pan of salted water to boil.
- Add the potato wedges to the pan of boiling water let boil for 8 minutes.
- Drain any excess water in a colander, let steam dry for briefly.
- Transfer to a roasting tray.
- Add olive oil together with a pinch of salt and pepper.
- Toss to coat the wedges with oil, spread out in one layer.
- Let cook in the hot oven for 30 minutes or until golden and cooked through.
- Serve and enjoy with chicken or a dip.

Brothy tortellini soup with spinach, white beans, and basil

Ingredients

- 1 can of white beans
- 2 tablespoons of <u>olive oil</u>
- 8 ounces of chopped baby spinach
- 1 onion, diced
- 6 garlic cloves, rough chopped
- 1 teaspoon of <u>salt</u>
- 1 cup of fresh basil, chopped
- ½ teaspoon of pepper
- 1 cup of celery, diced
- 10 ounces of fresh tortellini
- 8 cups of veggie
- Squeeze of lemon
- 1 teaspoon of dry Italian herbs

Directions

- Begin by heating olive oil in a large heavy bottom pot over medium-high heat.
- Add the onion to sauté for 4 minutes, stirring.

- Add the celery with garlic, lower heat to medium, let sauté for 6 minutes until celery is tender.
- Add the broth, then raise the heat to high, bring to a boil.
- Season with <u>salt</u> and Italian seasoning.
- Add the fresh tortellini when boiling, let simmer for 5 minutes or until cooked.
- Add the white beans and simmer briefly until heated through.
- Add the chopped fresh spinach together with the basil, after turning off the heat.
- Stir, and add a little squeeze of lemon.
- Taste, and adjust the seasoning.
- Serve and enjoy with a drizzle of <u>olive oil</u> , <u>pecorino</u> cheese and a light sprinkle of chili flakes.

Vegan ramen with shiitake broth

Ingredients

- 2 tablespoons of white <u>miso</u> paste
- 1 large onion-diced
- Pepper to taste
- 2 smashed garlic cloves
- Sriracha to taste
- 2 tablespoon of <u>olive oil</u>
- 8 ounces of <u>Ramen Noodles</u>
- 4 cups of <u>veggie stock</u>
- 8 ounces of cubed crispy tofu
- 4 cups of water
- ½ cup of <u>dried Shiitake</u> Mushrooms
- 1 sheet <u>Kombu</u> seaweed
- 1/8 cup of <u>mirin</u>

Directions

- **Sauté onion o** ver medium-high heat in 1 tablespoon olive oil until tender about 3 minutes.

- Turn heat to medium, add the smashed garlic cloves, let the onions cook until deeply golden brown.
- Add the veggie stock with water, dried shiitakes, a sheet of kombu , and mirin . Let Simmer for 30 minutes uncovered.
- R *emove the* Kombu .
- Then, add the miso with pepper to taste.
- In a pot of boiling water, cook the ramen noodles according to directions. Drain.
- Toss with sesame oil to keep separated.
- **Sauté the spinach and** mushrooms in olive oil until tender.
- Seasoning with salt and pepper.
- Fill bowls with cooked noodles, crispy tofu , and any other veggies.
- Pour the flavorful Shiitake broth over top.
- Serve and enjoy garnished with srirachi.

Cornbread casserole

Ingredients

- 2 large eggs
- 2 tablespoons of olive oil
- 1 cup of sour cream
- 1 onion, diced
- ¼ cup of melted butter
- 1 red bell pepper, diced
- 2 teaspoons of baking powder
- 4 cups of corn
- 1 ½ cups of grated cheese cheddar
- 4-ounce can of diced green chilies
- 1 teaspoon of cumin
- 1 teaspoon of coriander
- Salt
- 2 tablespoons chopped cilantro
- ½ cup of cornmeal
- 1 teaspoon of smoked paprika
- ½ cup of all-purpose flour
- 2 teaspoon of sugar

Directions

- In a large skillet, over medium heat, sauté onion in <u>olive oil</u> until fragrant in 4 minutes.
- Add the bell pepper, let cook for 4 minutes.
- Add the fresh corn and let sauté for 4 minutes.
- Stir in fresh cilantro.
- In a large bowl, combine cornmeal together with the salt, flour, baking powder, and sugar, whisk.
- In a separate medium bowl, whisk eggs with the sour cream. Then, gently whisk in the melted butter.
- Add the sautéed corn/pepper mixture to the dry ingredients with the egg mixture, stir to combine.
- Add 3/4 cup of grated cheese.
- Pour the batter into the greased baking dish.
- Topping with the remaining 3/4 cup of cheese.
- Bake for 35 minutes uncovered.
- Serve and enjoy warm sprinkled with cilantro.

Thai green curry

Ingredients

- Lime wedges for garnish
- ½ cup of homemade green curry paste
- 1 Japanese eggplant
- 1 teaspoon of sugar
- 2 tablespoons of olive oil
- 8 kefir lime leaves
- 1 cup of chicken broth
- ¼ cup of fresh Thai basil leaves, torn
- 1 can of coconut milk
- 8 ounces' pound of extra-firm tofu, cubed
- ½ teaspoon of salt
- 2 teaspoons of fish sauce
- 1 red bell pepper, sliced
- Lime juice to taste

Directions

- Begin by heating olive oil in a heavy bottom pot over medium-high heat.
- Stir-fry the homemade green curry paste for 3 minutes.

- Add the stock, then Stir in one can of full coconut milk .
- Add salt , sugar , and fish sauce
- Add the tofu together with the veggies and kefir lime leaves.
- Bring to a gentle simmer, uncovered until eggplant softens.
- Add a squeeze of lime and taste, and adjust accordingly.
- Add the fresh basil leaves and serve with lime wedges over rice.
- Enjoy.

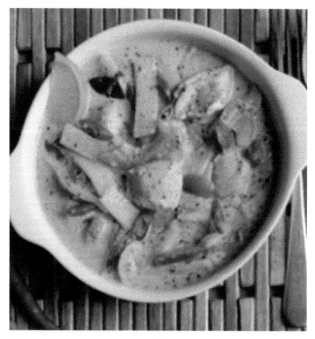

Kimchi burritos

Ingredients

- 1 cup of shredded cheese
- ½ cup of kimchi , chopped
- 2 tablespoon of olive oil
- 2 scallions, chopped
- 1 onion, diced
- Cilantro, hot sauce
- Salt to taste
- 1 red bell pepper, diced
- 1 cup of rice
- 1 can of black beans, rinsed, strained

Directions

- In a large skillet, heat oil over medium heat.
- Then, sauté onion with bell pepper for 5 minutes or until tender.
- Add rice together with kimchi and black beans, stir to combine.
- Season with salt and scallions.
- Taste, and adjust spices accordingly.

- Add cheese to the pan, gently melt, stirring for until melty and stringy.

- Divide filling into the center of the warm tortillas.

- Top with <u>hot sauce</u> and or cilantro and wrap into a burrito.

- Serve and enjoy immediately.

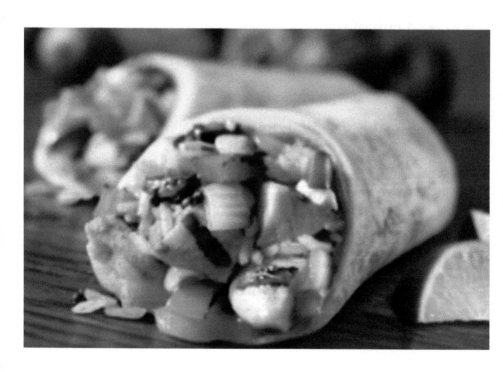

Singapore style fried rice

This specific Mediterranean Sea diet recipe has many variations with a perfect seasoning and fluffiness, if can be blended with various vegetables of your liking.

Ingredients

- 1 teaspoon of chili jam
- 4 fresh or frozen raw peeled prawns
- 150g of brown
- 1 teaspoon of mixed seeds
- 320g of crunchy veggies
- 1 tablespoon of low-salt soy sauce
- 1 teaspoon of tikka paste
- 1 rasher of smoked streaky bacon
- 1 clove of garlic
- 2cm of piece of ginger
- 1 large free-range egg
- Olive oil
- 1 chipolata

Directions

- Start by cooking the rice according as per packet Directions.

- Drain any excess water let cool.
- Put a large non-stick frying pan on a medium-high heat.
- Place 1 teaspoon of olive oil into the hot pan.
- Pour in the egg, swirl around the pan.
- Cook through, remove and roll up and slice.
- Put ½ a tablespoon of olive oil into the hot pan.
- Stir-fry the bacon with sausages until golden.
- Add the prawns with garlic and ginger.
- Stir in the curry paste to coated everything.
- Add the vegetables, begin with hard to cook veggies. Keep stirring.
- Place in the cool rice and stir-fry until the veggies are just cooked.
- Add the soy, toss in the egg ribbons.
- Divide between plates, sprinkle over the seeds.
- Season and adjust accordingly.
- Serve and enjoy with a drizzle of chili jam.

Purple cauliflower salad

Ingredients

- 2 tablespoons of <u>red wine vinegar</u>
- ½ cup of Italian parsley, chopped
- 1 head cauliflower
- ½ teaspoon of pepper
- 2 cloves garlic, minced
- Salt
- zest of one lemon
- 2 cups of cooked grain- <u>black rice</u>
- 2 scallions, sliced
- ½ cup of sliced Kalamata olives
- 2 tablespoons of <u>capers</u>
- <u>olive oil</u>

Directions

- Preheat your oven to 425°F.
- Set grains to cook on the stove.
- Remove and let cool.
- Cut cauliflower into bite-sized florets.
- Then, slightly toss in <u>olive oil</u> , <u>salt</u> and lemon zest.

- Spread out on a <u>parchment</u> -lined baking sheet.
- Let roast for 25 minutes, turning halfway through. Let cool.
- In a bowl, whisk olive oil, red wine vinegar, garlic, salt, and pepper.
- Layer salad ingredients in a shallow bowl starting with the grain.
- Serve and enjoy.

Grilled cabbage with andouille sausage

Ingredients

- 1 tablespoon of <u>olive oil</u>
- 1 tablespoon of fresh chives
- 2 tablespoons of <u>whole grain mustard</u>
- 1 ½ tablespoons of <u>honey</u>
- 1 large purple cabbage
- <u>Olive oil</u> for brushing
- Salt and pepper
- 6 andouille sausages
- ¼ teaspoon of <u>salt</u>
- ¼ teaspoon of pepper
- 2 tablespoons of <u>apple cider vinegar</u>

<u>Directions</u>

- Preheat your <u>grill</u> on high heat.
- Grease the <u>grill</u> well.
- Brush each side of cabbage with <u>olive oil</u> .
- Season with <u>salt</u> and pepper.
- lower <u>grill</u> to medium heat, then add sausages and thinly sliced cabbage.
- <u>Grill</u> the cabbage for 8 minutes on both sides.

- <u>Grill</u> the sausages until seared.
- Place cabbage steaks down on a large platter.
- Spoon half of the dressing over top.
- Slice the sausages in half and steep diagonal and scatter over cabbage.
- Serve and enjoy garnished with chopped chives.

Superfood walnut pesto noodles

Ingredients

- ¼ cup of sliced radishes
- 1 cup of walnuts
- ¼ cup of walnuts
- 2 tablespoons of <u>sesame oil</u>
- 4 ounces of dry <u>soba noodles</u>
- 1 cup of power greens
- Squeeze of lemon to taste
- 2 tablespoons of white <u>miso</u>
- <u>Olive oil</u> and lemon for drizzling
- 2 garlic cloves, start with one
- ¼ cup water
- 4 cups of baby superfood greens
- ½ cup of shredded cabbage
- Edamame, sunflower sprouts, <u>avocado</u> , snow peas

Directions

- Cook soba noodles according to the package ins

- Place walnuts together with the <u>miso</u>, olive oil, garlic, and water into a food processor, blend repeatedly.
- Then, add the power greens and pulse.
- Taste and adjust the taste and consistence.
- Toss the noodles with walnut pesto.
- Place noodles in a bento box with a handful of greens, shredded cabbage, walnuts, and radishes.
- Drizzle vegetables with a little <u>olive oil</u>, lemon, and <u>salt</u>.
- Serve and enjoy.

Carrots soup with chermoula

Ingredients

- ½ a large onion
- 1 tablespoon of lemon juice
- 1 ½ teaspoon of Cumin seeds
- ¼ teaspoon of salt
- 4 garlic cloves, smashed
- 4 cups chicken stock
- 2 bay leaves
- Zest from ½ lemon
- 1 teaspoon of kosher salt
- ¼ teaspoon of white pepper
- ¼ teaspoon of chili flakes
- 2 teaspoons of honey
- ¼ cup of yogurt
- 1 teaspoon of cumin seeds , toasted
- 1 lbs. carrots, cut into disks
- 1 teaspoon of fresh thyme
- 1 teaspoon coriander seeds, toasted
- 1 cup of cilantro
- ½ cup of Italian parsley

- 1 teaspoon of fresh ginger
- 2 garlic cloves
- Olive oil

Directions

- Sauté onion together with the <u>cumin seeds</u> and smashed garlic in olive oil over medium high heat until golden, stirring often.
- Add carrots with chicken stock, bay leaves, <u>salt</u> , <u>white pepper</u> .
- Bring to a vigorous simmer, lower, simmer covered for 20 minutes over low heat.
- Then, toast the spices in a dry skillet over medium heat until fragrant.
- Combine all ingredients in a <u>food processor</u> , blend to form paste. Keep aside for later.
- Blend the soup using an immersion blender or in small batches.
- Place back in the pot, stir in sour cream and <u>maple syrup</u> .
- Taste, and adjust seasoning.
- Divide among bowls, then add a spoonful of chermoula, swirl in a circle.

- Serve and enjoy.

Lemony corona beans with olive and garlic

Ingredients

- Salt and pepper to taste
- 2 teaspoons of <u>kosher salt</u>
- ¼ cup of fresh parsley leaves
- 2 bay leaves
- 3 celery sticks, cut into pieces
- <u>Aleppo</u> chili flakes
- 1 onion, quartered
- zest of one lemon
- 1 lb. dry <u>Royal Corona Beans</u>
- 4 garlic cloves, smashed
- A few fresh sage leaves
- 3 tablespoons of <u>olive oil</u>

<u>Directions</u>

- Place soaked beans in a large <u>Dutch oven</u> with water enough to cover them.
- Add <u>salt</u> together with the celery, garlic, onion, bay leaves, and herbs.

- Bring to a boil, lower heat, let simmer covered until tender n about 2 hours.
- Drain, reserve some liquid without the aromatics for later.
- Place in a <u>serving dish</u> .
- Then, add back 1 cup of the reserved warm cooking liquid with <u>olive oil</u> , lemon zest, fresh Italian parsley, and <u>salt</u> and pepper.
- Serve and enjoy.

Szechuan tofu and vegetables

Ingredients

- 1 cup of asparagus, snap peas
- 12 ounces of tofu, patted dry, cubed
- ¼ cup of Szechuan Sauce
- 1 cup of shredded carrots
- 2 tablespoons of peanut oil
- generous pinch of salt and pepper
- ½ red bell pepper, thinly sliced
- ½ cup of thinly sliced onion
- Scallions of sesame seeds
- 4 ounces of sliced mushrooms
- 2 cups of shredded cabbage

Directions

- Heat olive oil in a skillet over medium heat.
- Season peanut oil together with salt and pepper.
- Then, swirl the seasoned peanut oil to spread out uniformly.
- Add tofu and sear on at least two sides, until crispy and golden.

- In the same pan, add onion and mushrooms.
- Sauté over medium-high heat, stirring constantly, until tender.
- Add the remaining vegetables with dried red chilies
- Lower heat to medium, sauté, while tossing and stirring for 5 minutes.
- Add the Szechuan Sauce , gradually.
- Let cook for 2 minutes, until thickened a bit.
- Toss in the crispy tofu towards the end.
- Divide among bowls.
- Sprinkle with sesame seeds and scallions.
- Serve and enjoy with noodles or over rice.

Kyoto roasted sweet potatoes with miso, ginger, and scallions

Ingredients

- Salt to taste
- 3 yams sliced in half
- 2 teaspoons of ginger finely minced
- 3 Scallions, sliced
- Olive oil for brushing
- 1 tablespoon of <u>miso</u>
- ¼ cup of <u>olive oil</u>
- 1 large shallot, finely diced

Directions

- Preheat your oven ready to 425°F.
- Place cut sweet potatoes on a <u>parchment</u> -lined <u>sheet pan</u>
- Brush with <u>olive oil</u> .
- Let roast for 40 minutes until fork tender.
- Heat the olive oil over medium low heat.
- Then, add the shallot to sauté until golden, stirring often.

- Add the ginger, continue to cook for 3 more minutes.
- Add and mash the <u>miso</u> with a fork into the mixture. Turn off the heat.
- After the sweet potatoes are caramelized, remove and place on a platter flesh side up.
- Reheat the miso, pierce the flesh in a few spots, spoon a tablespoon of the sauce over each one with the flavor.
- Sprinkle with a little <u>finishing salt</u> and scallions.
- Serve and enjoy.

Lemon sole with chipotle and ancho chili recado

Ingredients

- 1 ripe avocado
- Extra virgin olive oil
- 2 limes
- 4 cloves of garlic
- 2 dried chipotle chilies
- 3 spring onions
- 2 dried ancho chilies
- 1½ tablespoon of dried oregano
- 4 lemon sole
- ½ a lime
- 14 ripe cherry tomatoes
- 1 Lebanese cucumber

Directions

- Preheat the oven ready to 380°F.
- Place the unpeeled garlic in a small roasting tin and roast for 20 minutes.
- Transfer to a plate, let cool, then remove the skins.

- Place the chipotle together with the ancho chilies in a small bowl.
- Pour over boiling water to just cover, let soak for 15 minutes.
- Drain in a colander, reserving some liquid.
- Place the chilies together with the garlic, oregano, and a large pinch of sea salt in a food processor and blend to a paste.
- Add the lime juice and 4 tablespoons of the reserved liquid, blend further to combine.
- Transfer to a non-reactive bowl.
- Place the fish in the marinade, cover with Clingfilm.
- Refrigerate for 30 minutes.
- Combine chopped cucumber, spring onions, tomatoes, an avocado in a bowl with 3 tablespoons of oil and the lime juice.
- Season.
- Preheat a barbecue to a medium heat.
- Remove the fish from the refrigerator and cook, turning once, for about 3 minutes each side, brushing with marinade during cooking.

- Serve and enjoy with the avocado salad and freshly squeezed lime wedges.

Salsa Verde fresco

Ingredients

- ½ a bunch of fresh coriander
- 2 large fresh green chilies
- 2 limes
- 12 green tomatillos
- 2 onions
- 1 ripe avocado
- 1 clove of garlic

Directions

- Heat a griddle pan until screaming hot.
- Then, chargrill the chilies until their skins are black and blistered all over.
- Place the charred chilies in a bowl, cover with Clingfilm, let sit for a few minutes.
- In batches, chargrill the tomatillos with onion wedges until blackened and caramelised on all sides.
- Remove the chilies from the bowl and peel off the blackened skin.

- Place the chilies together with the onions, garlic, tomatillos, coriander leaves, and avocado on a big board.
- Chop all vegetables, mix in the lime juice and a good pinch of sea salt and black pepper.
- Blend all the ingredients in a blender until smooth.
- Drip onto eggs or on crispy chicken.
- Serve and enjoy.

Chilled avocado soup with tortilla chips

Ingredients

- 1 handful of micro garlic chives
- ½ tablespoon of olive oil
- 1 cucumber
- 4 spring onions
- 200ml of plain yoghurt
- ½ teaspoon of hot smoked paprika
- A few sprigs of fresh coriander
- 2 soft corn tortillas
- 1 large ripe avocado
- 250ml of organic vegetable stock
- 1 mild fresh green chili
- 1 lime
- Tabasco sauce
- 1 fresh red chili

Directions

- Preheat the oven to 400°F.
- Combine the oil together with the paprika, brush over both sides of the tortillas.

- Bake on a baking tray for 5 minutes, or until golden.
- Season well and set aside to cool, break into pieces.
- Blend the avocado together with the cucumber, stock, yoghurt, spring onions, coriander, and green chili until smooth.
- Then, season with lime juice, Tabasco, and a good pinch of sea salt and black pepper.
- Cover and place in the fridge to chill.
- Once the soup is chilled, serve in small bowls topped with the tortilla chips, chopped cucumber, red chili and garlic chives.
- Serve and enjoy with a drizzle of avocado oil.

Charred avocado and eggs

Ingredients

- ½ of a fresh red chili
- 4 spring onions
- A few sprigs of fresh soft herbs
- 2 tablespoons of cottage cheese
- ½ a ripe avocado
- Olive oil
- 1 sweet potato
- 1 red pepper
- 2 large free-range eggs

Directions

- Heat 1 tablespoon of olive oil over a medium-high heat.
- Add the spring onions together with the avocado and pepper, let fry for 4 minutes, or until lightly charred.
- Add peeled potatoes to the pan, toss with the charred vegetables, let fry for 3 minutes.
- Spread the vegetables evenly in the pan.
- Dig out 2 pockets.

- Crack an egg into each one, then tilt the pan so the whites run into the vegetables binding everything together.
- Season with sea salt and black pepper.
- Cover, with tin foil, lower the heat to medium–low, let the eggs cook for 5 minutes.
- Spoon the mixture onto a plate, dollop with cottage cheese and sprinkle over the herbs.

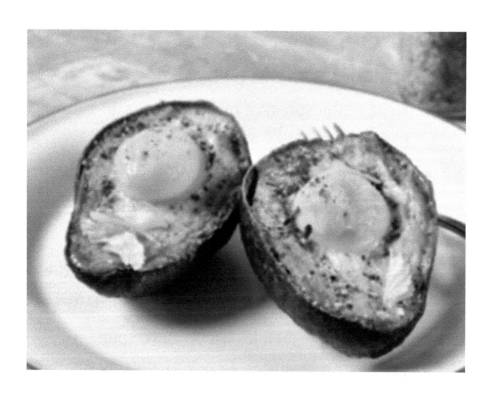

Avocado and slow roasted tomatoes on the toast

Ingredients

- 4 handfuls of rocket
- 4 plum tomatoes
- 4 slices of sourdough bread
- Olive oil
- 150g of feta cheese
- 1 bunch of fresh basil
- 1 lemon
- 3 ripe avocados

Directions

- Preheat the oven to 280°F.
- Place the tomatoes cut-side up on a baking tray.
- Season generously and drizzle with oil.
- Then, roast gently for 2 hours or until dried out.
- Pound basil leaves in a pestle and mortar with a pinch of sea salt until to foam paste.

- Pour in a good splash of oil and squeeze in the juice of ½ lemon.
- Place avocado flesh in a bowl, squeeze in the other lemon half.
- Season with salt and pepper.
- Mash with a fork to bring it all together.
- Toast the bread, then divide between 4 plates and generously spread on the avocado and top with the tomatoes.
- Serve and enjoy with crumbled feta.

Avocado ice cream

Ingredients

- 500ml of whole milk
- 200g of sugar
- 4 ripe avocados
- 2 vanilla pods
- 1 lime
- 1 lemon

Directions

- Add vanilla to saucepan with the pods.
- Add the sugar with the zest and juice.
- Bring to the boil, let simmer for a couple of minutes to dissolve the sugar.
- Remove from heat, pour into a bowl, let cool.
- Once the syrup is cool, remove the vanilla pods.
- Blend the avocado flesh with the milk to a smooth, light consistency.
- Pour it into a large baking dish, place in a freezer.

- Whisk every half hour or so until frozen and smooth.
- Serve and enjoy.

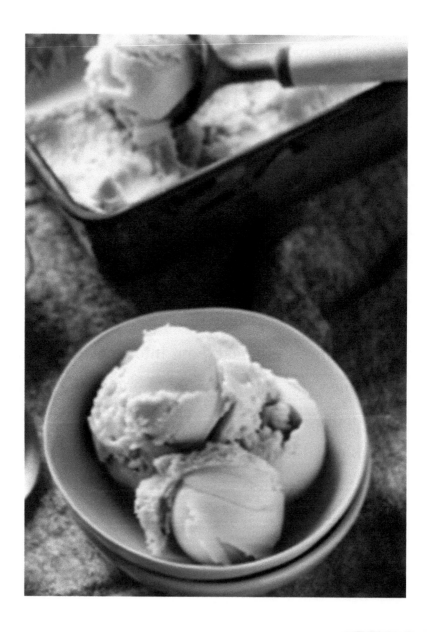

Quick flatbreads with avocado and feta

Ingredients

- 2 ripe avocados
- 250g of whole meal self-rising flour
- 1 teaspoon of rose harissa
- ¾ teaspoon of baking powder
- 75g of feta cheese
- 1 teaspoon cumin seeds
- 350g of plain yoghurt
- Olive oil

Directions

- Begin by toasting the cumin lightly in a dry pan, place in a bowl.
- Add the flour together with the baking powder, and yogurt.
- Season, and mix until dough forms.
- Turn out onto a lightly floured surface and knead until the dough together.
- Place in a lightly greased bowl, cover with a damp tea towel, let raise.

- Chop the avocado into chunks, then place in a bowl.
- Crumble in the feta with a drizzle of oil, season to taste.
- In another bowl, stir the harissa into the rest of the yoghurt.
- Divide the dough into eight balls.
- Roll each one on a lightly floured surface into an oval shape.
- Place a griddle pan over a high heat.
- Griddle each flatbread for 3 minutes, until puffed up.
- Brush the flatbread with a little oil.
- Serve and enjoy with the avocado salad and harissa yoghurt.

Smashed avocado, basil, and chicken

Ingredients

- 50g of leftover cooked chicken
- ½ of a ripe avocado
- Extra virgin olive oil
- 2 sprigs of fresh basil

Directions

- Place the avocado in a bowl and mash.
- Pick and tear in the basil leaves.
- Shred the chicken into small pieces.
- Add to the bowl.
- Then, Mix together, and add a little oil to loosen.
- Serve and enjoy.

Avocado, fig, and spinach

Ingredients

- 1 fresh fig
- ½ of a ripe avocado
- 1 large handful of baby spinach

Directions

- Place the avocado flesh in a blender.
- Add the spinach together with the fig.
- Blend to a purée.
- Taste, and adjust the thickness.
- Serve and enjoy.

Cracking cob salad

Ingredients

- 1 large pinch of sweet smoked paprika
- 2 tablespoons of Greek yoghurt
- Olive oil
- 4 slices of pancetta
- 2 large free-range eggs
- 2 free-range chicken thighs
- Extra virgin olive oil
- 1 Romaine, cos lettuce
- ½ teaspoon of Worcestershire sauce
- 1 ripe avocado
- 50ml of buttermilk
- 1 lemon
- 2 ripe tomatoes
- 1 punnet of salad cress
- 50g of Stilton
- ½ a bunch of fresh chives

Directions

- Preheat the oven to 350°F.

- Place the chicken thighs into a small roasting tray.
- Sprinkle over the paprika, and a pinch of sea salt and black pepper.
- Drizzle over a little olive oil and toss to coat.
- Let roast for 40 minutes, or until golden, laying over the pancetta for the final 10 minutes. Let cool slightly.
- Lower the eggs into a pan of vigorously simmering water and boil for 6 minutes, refreshing under cold water, peel.
- Crumble the Stilton into a large jug.
- Add chopped chives, with a drizzle of extra virgin olive oil.
- Squeeze in the lemon juice with the remaining dressing ingredients, whisk.
- Season to taste with salt and pepper, refrigerate until needed.
- Remove and discard any tatty outer leaves from the lettuce, chop the rest.
- Chop avocado, tomatoes, peeled eggs on a board and mix it together.

- Shred the chicken meat, without bones and skin.
- Add to the salad.
- Crumble over the crispy pancetta and continue chopping and mixing together.
- Transfer the salad to a platter, drizzle over the blue cheese dressing.
- Serve and enjoy.

Avocado and peas with mashed potato

Ingredients

- 1 sprig of fresh mint
- 1 potato
- 1 large ripe avocado
- 1 tablespoon of milk
- 100g of frozen peas

Directions

- Peel and dice the potato.
- Cook in boiling water for 10 minutes.
- Drain any excess water and mash with the milk.
- Cook the peas in boiling water for 3 minutes.
- Drain excess water, place into a bowl, let cool.
- Add chopped avocado to the bowl.
- Add the mint leaves and mash together.
- Serve and enjoy.

Avocado, pancetta, and pine nut salad

Ingredients

- 6 ripe avocados
- Sea salt
- 12 slices pancetta
- 50g of pine nuts
- Balsamic vinegar
- Freshly ground black pepper
- 4 big handfuls of baby spinach
- Extra virgin olive oil

Directions

- Heat a frying pan and fry the pancetta slices till crispy.
- Remove from the pan and set aside.
- In the same pan, lightly toast the pine nuts.
- Combining balsamic vinegar with olive oil.
- Season with salt and pepper.
- Lay out the avocado on a serving plate.
- Sprinkle over the spinach leaves, pancetta, and toasted pine nuts.

- Season with salt and pepper and drizzle over your dressing.
- Serve and enjoy with warm crusty bread.

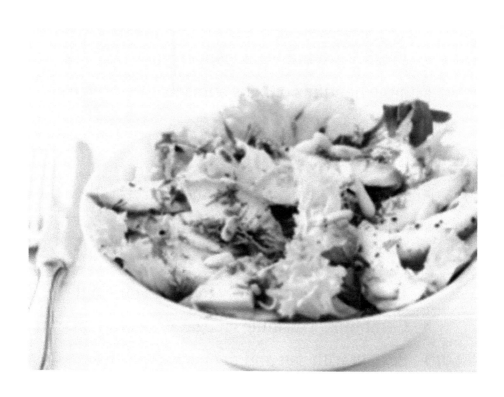

Roast carrot and avocado salad with orange and lemon dressing

Ingredients

- 2 handfuls of mixed winter salad leaves
- 500g of medium differently colored carrots
- 2 punnet cress
- 1 lemon
- 2 level teaspoons of whole cumin seeds
- 150ml of fat-free natural yoghurt
- 2 small dried chilies
- 3 ripe avocados
- 4 tablespoons of mixed seeds
- 2 cloves garlic
- Red wine vinegar
- 4 sprigs fresh thyme
- 4 x 1cm of thick slices ciabatta
- Extra virgin olive oil
- red or white wine vinegar
- 1 orange

Directions

- Preheat the oven to 350°F.

- Boil the carrots in boiling, salted water for 10 minutes.
- Drain, place into a roasting tray.
- Mash up the cumin seeds, chilies, salt and pepper in a mortar.
- Add the garlic with thyme leaves, smash up again until paste foams.
- Add enough extra virgin olive oil with vinegar to cover the past.
- Stir together, then pour over the carrots in the tray, to coat.
- Add the orange and lemon halves, cut-side down.
- Place in the preheated oven for 30 minutes.
- Remove the carrots, then add to the avocados.
- Squeeze the roasted orange and lemon juice into a bowl and add the same amount of extra virgin olive oil, with a swig of red wine vinegar.
- Season, and pour this dressing over the carrots and avocados.
- Mix together, taste and adjust the seasoning.

- Tear the toasted bread into little pieces and add to the dressed carrot and avocado.
- Serve and enjoy.

Smoked salmon and avocado salad

Ingredients

- Freshly ground black pepper
- 2 small avocados
- 1 lemon
- 200g of smoked salmon
- Sea salt
- ½ cucumber
- 2 handfuls of mixed fresh herbs
- 1 punnet cress
- 2 tablespoons of mixed seeds
- 1 loaf ciabatta
- 1 blood orange
- Extra virgin olive oil

Directions

- Heat a griddle pan until screaming hot.
- Place the sliced avocado in a bowl, squeeze over some lemon juice.
- Slice the cucumber into long, thin strips on top of the avocado.
- Then, add the herbs and cress.

- Lightly toast the seeds in a dry pan on a medium to low heat.
- Squeeze a tablespoon of juice out of the blood orange into a bowl.
- Add 3 tablespoons of extra virgin olive oil.
- Season. Mix.
- Place the ciabatta squares in the griddle pan, charring both sides.
- Once toasted, drizzle with a little of the dressing and put to one side.
- Place a square of ciabatta on each of four plates, then top each with a quarter of the smoked salmon.
- Drizzle the dressing over the salad and mix with your fingertips.
- Top the smoked salmon with the salad.
- Serve and enjoy.

Grilled chicken with charred pineapple salad

Ingredients

- ¼ of a pineapple
- ½ of an avocado
- 1 teaspoon of dried oregano
- ½ a bunch of fresh coriander
- Olive oil
- 1 fresh red chili
- 2 x 150g of free-range chicken breasts
- 2 tablespoons of pickled jalapeños
- 150 g quinoa
- 50g of white cabbage
- 2 limes
- 1 large handful of salad leaves
- 50g of natural yoghurt

Directions

- Begin by combining the oregano with olive oil in a bowl.
- Season with sea salt and black pepper.

- Place the chicken breast with olive oil in the bowl, turning until coated, then leave to one side.
- Then, cook the quinoa as per the packet Directions, drain, set aside.
- Place avocado flesh, coriander, jalapeno, and a splash of the pickling liquid and the juice of 1½ limes in a blender.
- Blend until smooth, stir through the quinoa.
- Place a griddle pan over a high heat.
- Place chopped apple on the hot griddle pan for a few minutes on each side.
- Transfer to a chopping board.
- In the same pan, griddle the chicken for 5 minutes on each side.
- Place on the chopping board, let rest and cool.
- Chop the griddled pineapple into bite-sized chunks, and the chili, then slice the chicken into thin strips.
- Divide the yoghurt among 4 plates topping with the chicken, and pineapple on one side and the dressed quinoa on the other.

- Toss the leaves and cabbage with the juice of the remaining lime, chopped chili and a little salt and pepper.
- Serve and enjoy.

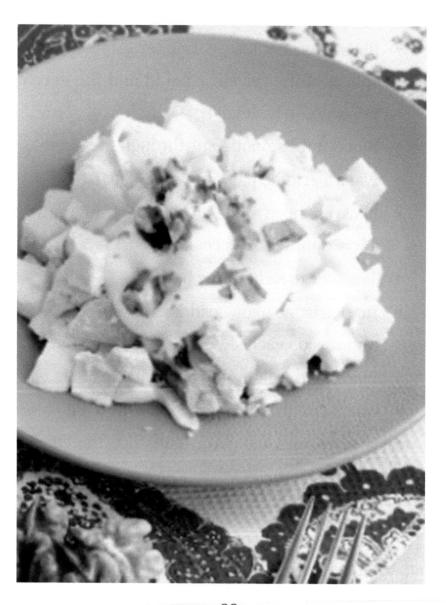

Salina chicken

Ingredients

- 4 sprigs of fresh basil
- 2 red onions
- 3 aubergines
- 1 x 1.4 kg whole free-range chicken
- olive oil
- 200g of ripe cherry tomatoes
- 2 cloves of garlic
- 3 small fresh red chilies
- 50g of pine nuts
- 2 lemons
- 1 cinnamon stick
- 4 sprigs of fresh woody herbs
- 50g of baby capers in brine

Directions

- Preheat the oven to 350°F.
- Place chopped aubergines in a large bowl.
- Then, season with sea salt.

- Drizzle the chicken pieces with olive oil, place in a large shallow pan on a medium-high heat, with skin side down turning to get golden.
- Wipe off the salt on aubergines and add to the pan, turning until lightly golden.
- Remove.
- Combine garlic with chilies, cinnamon, capers, and woody herbs add to the pan.
- Stir and fry for briefly, stir in onion, let cook for 15 minutes, stirring occasionally.
- Squeeze the tomatoes in a bowl of water, remove the seeds.
- Put the chicken and aubergines back in, drizzle over any resting juices, with half liter of water.
- Sprinkle over the pine nuts, then squeeze over the lemon juice.
- Cook at the bottom of the oven until golden.
- Pick over the basil leaves.
- Serve and enjoy with lemony couscous.

Chicken tikka skewers

Ingredients

- 3 fresh red chilies
- 2 lemons
- ½ a bunch of fresh coriander
- 2 teaspoons of tikka masala spice paste
- 2 tablespoons of natural yoghurt
- 2 little gem lettuces
- Olive oil
- ½ of a small ripe pineapple
- 2 skinless free-range chicken breasts

Directions

- Combine lemon juice, olive oil, paste, and yogurt, then mix well.
- Add sliced pineapple, chilies, sliced chicken to the bowl with the marinade.
- Toss together to coat, place in the fridge to marinate overnight.
- Remove the chicken and pineapple mixture from the fridge.
- Remove and tear the chili into smaller pieces.

- Starting with the chicken, thread the ingredients onto skewers, alternating between the ingredients.
- Pour any remaining marinade over the top and drizzle with a little oil.
- Put a dry pan on a medium heat, then add the skewers, let cook for 10 minutes, turning occasionally, season with a little sea salt.
- Roughly shave the chicken, pineapple and chili from the skewers with a knife, scatter over the reserved lemon zest and pick over the coriander leaves.
- Slice the remaining lemon into wedges for squeezing over.
- Serve and enjoy with the lettuce and yoghurt.

Sticky hoisin chicken

Ingredients

- 3 regular oranges
- 2 x 200g of free-range chicken legs
- 2 heaped tablespoons of hoisin sauce
- 2 fresh mixed-color chilies
- 8 spring onions

Directions

- Preheat the oven ready to 350°F.
- Place an ovenproof frying pan on a high heat.
- Pull off the chicken skin, put both skin and legs into the pan.
- Season with sea salt and black pepper, letting the fat render out and the chicken get golden, turning halfway.
- Toss the white spring onions into the pan, after which transfer to the oven for 15 minutes.
- Place chilies and green spring onions into a bowl of ice-cold water to curl.
- Arrange sliced oranges on a plates.

- Remove the chicken skin and soft spring onions from the pan. Set aside.
- Cook the chicken until tender and cooked through.
- In a bowl, loosen the hoisin with a splash of red wine vinegar, spoon over the chicken.
- Sit the chicken and soft spring onions on top and crack over the crispy skin.
- Serve and enjoy.

Sweet chicken surprise

Ingredients

- 4 sprigs of fresh tarragon
- 2 x 200g of free-range chicken legs
- 100ml of red vermouth
- 1 bulb of garlic
- 250g of mixed-color seedless grapes

Directions

- Start by preheating the oven to 350°F.
- Then, place an ovenproof frying pan over high heat.
- Rub the chicken with ½ a tablespoon of olive oil.
- Then, season with sea salt and black pepper and place skin side down in the pan.
- Fry for a couple of minutes until golden.
- Squash the unpeeled garlic cloves, add with grapes to the pan.
- Turn the chicken skin side up, then pour in the vermouth.

- Transfer to the oven, let roast for 40 minutes, or until the chicken tender.
- Add a splash of water to the pan and to pick up all the sticky bits.
- Serve and enjoy.

Sesame butterflied chicken

Ingredients

- 2 tablespoons of natural yoghurt
- 1 tablespoon of low-salt soy sauce
- 100g of fine rice noodles
- 2cm piece of ginger
- 2 x 120g of skinless free-range chicken breasts
- 1 tablespoon of peanut butter
- 2 teaspoons of sesame seeds
- 2 limes
- Groundnut oil
- 4 spring onions
- ½ of a Chinese cabbage
- 200g of sugar snap peas
- 1 fresh red chili

Directions

- Place your griddle pan over high heat.
- Then, in a bowl, cover the noodles with boiling kettle water.
- Rub with 1 teaspoon of groundnut oil on chicken opened up.

- Season with a small pinch of sea salt and black pepper.
- Let griddle for 8 minutes, turning halfway.
- Trim the spring onions and rattle them through the finest slicer on your food processor with the Chinese cabbage, sugar snap peas and chili.
- Dress with the juice of 1 lime and the soy sauce.
- In a separate small bowl, mix the peanut butter together with the yoghurt and the juice of the remaining lime, ginger, mix.
- Slice the chicken on a board, toast lightly with the sesame seeds in the residual heat of the griddle pan.
- Sprinkle over the chicken.
- Drain the noodles, divide between plates with the chicken, slaw and peanut sauce, mix.
- Serve and enjoy.

Chicken and spring green bun cha

Ingredients

- ½ a bunch of fresh mint
- 2 spring onions
- 100g frozen edamame beans
- 1 stick of lemongrass
- 3 tablespoons of vegetable oil
- 5cm piece of ginger
- 1 large fresh red chili
- 200g of baby spinach
- 1½ tablespoons of sesame oil
- 1 tablespoon of low-salt soy sauce
- 150g of broad beans
- 2 tablespoons of runny honey
- 2 tablespoons of hoisin sauce
- 2 limes
- 4 free-range skinless chicken thighs
- 1 tablespoon of rice wine vinegar
- 1 x 225g packet of vermicelli
- 2 large shallots
- ½ a bunch of fresh Thai basil

Directions

- Preheat the oven to 400°F.
- Place the lemongrass in a large bowl together with the sesame oil, soy sauce, the zest from 1 lime, honey, hoisin sauce, and the juice from 2 limes. Mix, pour half into a small bowl.
- Add the chicken to the large bowl, stir and let marinate.
- Add the rice wine vinegar to the small bowl.
- Cook defrosted beans in a pan of boiling water for 2 minutes.
- Drain and rinse under cold water. Set aside.
- Cook the vermicelli according to the packet Directions, drain.
- Place the chicken in a small roasting tin lined with tinfoil, move it in the oven heated for 30 minutes.
- Then, heat olive oil in a small, pan over a medium-high heat.
- When hot enough, add the shallots, let cook for 5 minutes.

- Remove, set aside on a tray lined with kitchen paper.
- Combine the noodles together with the remaining dressing, spring onion, broad beans, baby spinach, and herbs.
- Top with the chicken, garnished with the shallots.
- Serve and enjoy.

Firecracker chicken noodle salad

Ingredients

- 1 tablespoon of sweet chili sauce
- 1 tablespoon of coriander oil
- 50g of rice noodles
- ½ tablespoon of low-salt soy sauce
- 1 lime
- 100g of cooked free-range chicken
- ¼ of a cucumber
- 1 carrot
- ½ tablespoon of runny honey
- 1 baby gem lettuce
- 1 small handful of sugar snaps
- A few sprigs of fresh mint
- 1 pinch of mixed seeds

Directions

- Cook the noodles as instructed on the package.
- Combine the shredded chicken with the cooked noodles and coriander oil in a bowl.
- Add all the remaining salad ingredients, toss to combine.

- Place the sweet chili sauce together with the soy and honey in a small jar. Chill in the lunchbox.
- Squeeze in the lime juice, secure the lid, keep in the lunchbox.
- Shake the jam jar to mix the ingredients then dress the salad.
- Close your lunchbox, shake to coat.
- Serve and enjoy chilled or at room temperature.

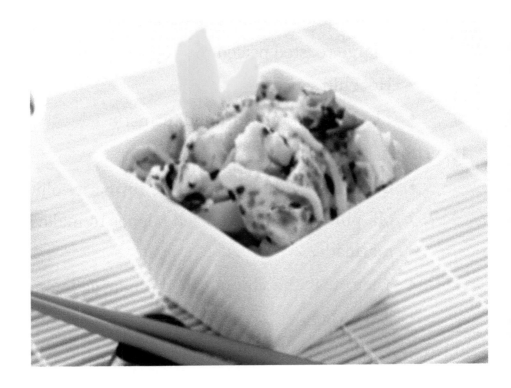

Seared turmeric chicken

Ingredients

- Olive oil
- 200g of seasonal greens
- 2 x 120g of skinless chicken breasts
- 150g of whole wheat couscous
- 2 tablespoons of natural yoghurt
- 2 sprigs of fresh oregano
- ½ a bunch of fresh mint
- 1 lemon
- 1 tablespoon of blanched hazelnuts
- 2 large roasted peeled red peppers in brine
- Hot chili sauce
- 1 level teaspoon of ground turmeric

Directions

- Combine the oregano leaves, turmeric, olive oil, pinch of salt and black pepper to make a marinade.
- Then, toss the chicken in the marinade and leave aside.

- In a boiling water, blanch the greens until tender enough to eat, drain, reserving the water.
- In a bowl, cover the couscous with boiling greens water, season with a plate on top for 10 minutes.
- Stir chopped mint leaves into the fluffy couscous with the juice of half a lemon.
- Toast the hazelnuts in a large dry frying pan on a medium-high heat.
- Remove, and crush in mortar once lightly golden.
- Return the frying pan to a high heat, let the chicken cook for 4 minutes on each side, turning halfway.
- Serve the chicken with the couscous, peppers, greens and yoghurt, scattered with the hazelnuts, with a lemon wedge on the side.
- Enjoy.

Chicken and garlic bread kebabs

Ingredients

- 1 lemon
- 2 sprigs of fresh rosemary
- 2 blood oranges
- 1 tablespoon of balsamic vinegar
- 2 cloves of garlic
- Extra virgin olive oil
- 1 tablespoon white wine vinegar
- 20g of feta cheese
- 8 fresh bay leaves
- Cayenne pepper
- 2 x 120g skinless chicken breasts
- 2 thick slices of whole meal bread
- 100g of baby spinach

Directions

- Mash up rosemary with a pinch of sea salt in a pestle and mortar. Peel and crush in the garlic, then muddle in 1 tablespoon of oil, the vinegar and a generous pinch of cayenne.

- Place chopped chicken and bread in a bowl, toss to mix well with the marinade until evenly coated.
- Place the frying pan on a medium-high heat.
- Then, lay the skewers in the pan, let cook for 5 minutes on each side.
- Dress the spinach with a squeeze of lemon juice and a drizzle of olive oil.
- Organize on the plates with the blood oranges and drizzle with the balsamic.
- Serve and enjoy topped with the kebabs and lemon wedges.

Piri piri chicken

Ingredients

- 1.3kg of chicken
- 3 sprigs of fresh thyme
- 4 cloves of garlic
- Olive oil
- 2 red onions
- 4 ripe mixed-color tomatoes
- 6 fresh mixed-color chilies
- Red wine vinegar
- Extra virgin olive oil
- 750g of sweet potatoes
- 2 teaspoons of smoked paprika
- 2 tablespoons of fine semolina
- 1 x 200g jar of pickled jalapeños
- 1 bunch of fresh coriander

Directions

- Combine thyme leaves, garlic, paprika, and a pinch of sea salt in a pestle and mortar.
- Blend to foam paste, add 2 tablespoons of olive oil.

- Rub the marinade on the chicken.
- Cover properly, and refrigerate to marinate overnight or more than, two hours, if one has no time.
- Preheat the oven to 350°F.
- Then, place a large griddle pan over a high heat.
- Place unpeeled onions and tomatoes, chilies, and unpeeled garlic on the hot griddle.
- Let, grill for 10 minutes, turning regularly.
- Remove the garlic skins and peel the onions.
- Add every vegetable to a food processor with a splash of red wine vinegar and extra virgin olive oil.
- Blend until smooth, adjusting with water if too thick.
- Season, and adjust.
- Return the griddle pan to a high heat, then add the marinated chicken and sear all over for 10 minutes, turning regularly.
- Then, transfer to a roasting tray, put in the hot oven for 45 minutes.

- Toss the sweet potatoes with the paprika, semolina, extra virgin olive oil, a small pinch of salt and black pepper.
- Spread the wedges out on 2 large baking trays.
- Place in the oven for 30 minutes, or until tender and crisp.
- Drain and add the jalapeños to a food processor with a splash of the pickling juice.
- Tear in the coriander with a splash of extra virgin olive oil.
- Blend until smooth.
- Serve the roast chicken with piri piri sauce, sweet potato wedges and a little jalapeño salsa.
- Enjoy.

Steaming ramen

Ingredients

- 8 chicken wings
- 1 handful of pork bones
- 200ml of low-salt soy sauce
- 2 sheets of wakame seaweed
- 750g of pork belly
- 2 thumb-sized pieces of ginger

Sesame oil

- 1 thumb-sized piece of ginger
- 1 splash of mirin
- 1 heaped tablespoon of miso paste
- 400g of baby spinach
- 500g of dried soba
- 8 tablespoons of kimchee
- 8 small handfuls of beansprouts
- 4-star anise
- 8 spring onions
- 7 garlic
- 2 fresh red chilies
- Chili oil

- 4 large free-range eggs

Directions

- Boil the eggs for 5 minutes.
- Pour the soy sauce, mirin, and star anise, with water into a small pan.
- Boil ginger and garlic, remove from the heat, then, pour the mixture into a sandwich bag with the eggs.
- Place in refrigerator for 6 hours, then drain.
- Preheat the oven to 400°F.
- Place chicken wings together with the pork bones into a large casserole pan.
- Bash, add the unpeeled ginger and garlic.
- Toss with a good drizzle of sesame oil.
- Place the pork skin on a baking tray, bake for around 40 minutes.
- Cover pork belly and miso with water, bring to the boil.
- Simmer over low heat for 3 hours, or until the pork belly is tender, skimming occasionally.
- Lift the pork belly onto a tray and put aside.

- Sieve the broth and pour back into the pan. Return to the heat and reduce the liquid down.
- Place a large colander over the pan and steam the spinach until wilted.
- In another separate pan, cook the noodles according to packet Directions, drain.
- Divide between 8 large warm bowls with the beansprouts and spinach.
- Taste the broth and adjust the seasoning.
- Tear over the seaweed and divide up the kimchee.

Serve and enjoy drizzle with chili oil.

Lightning Source UK Ltd.
Milton Keynes UK
UKHW020746030621
384855UK00001B/164